Lean And Green Diet crash course

The Succinct Guide To Healthy And Delicious Meals To Burn Fat Quickly, Regain The Fitness You Deserve Now And Get Back In Shape With The Fat-Burning Power Of Lean And Green Meals

Natalie Allen

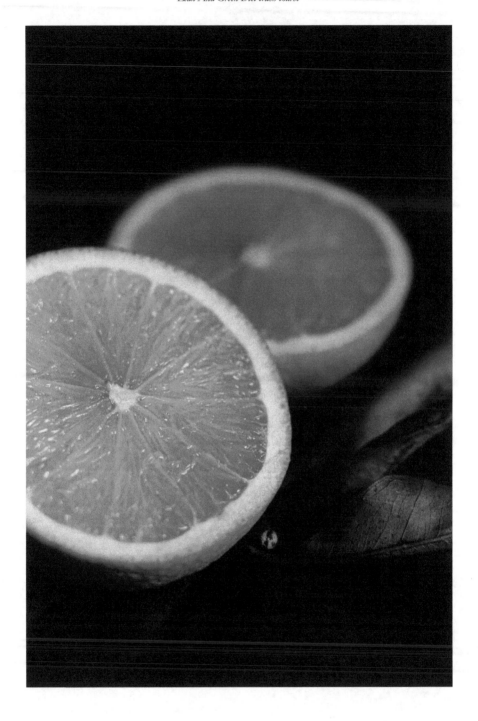

TABLE OF CONTENTS

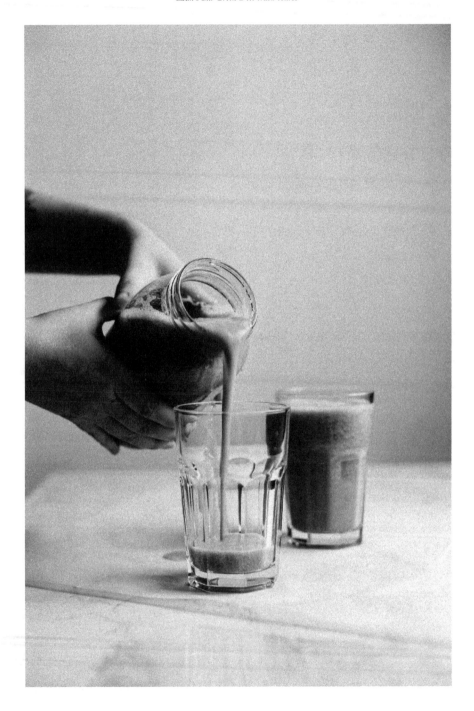

Introduction

One way is by changing your diet and cooking in a smarter way. Lean and Green Cookbook provides recipes for delicious, healthy food with reduced environmental impact. Get ready to cook up a storm that's good for the environment!

This article was written because there are so many people who want tips and tricks on how to stay lean while reducing their environmental impact. It does not matter if you are a novice or a pro chef; this book will educate and inspire a way to make the best out of the foods you eat. Eat healthy with dietary guidelines in mind. s

The cookbook is full of a little bit of everything from main dishes to light breakfasts. From protein-packed animal and seafood recipes to balanced and delicious vegetarian and vegan dishes. So, get ready for a feast on the go! You'll be amazed just how tasty healthy can be in a nutshell.

Lean and Green is perfect for people who want to cook healthy food without a lot of hassle or spending a lot of time in the kitchen. It includes easy recipes that take 30 minutes or less to make, making it ideal for busy people with hectic schedules. In addition, the book is also loaded with nutritional information about every recipe, including calories, fat, carbohydrates, and protein content.

Vegetarian Delicacies: Everything you need to know about vegetarian cuisine. These dishes include Mexican, Italian, Chinese, Indian, Thai, Greek, French, Japanese, and Taiwanese. The recipes are based on traditional food from these countries that are healthy without being bland or boring. These recipes are also vegan and gluten-free.

Everything you need to know about vegetarian cuisine. These dishes include Mexican, Italian, Chinese, Indian, Thai, Greek, French, Japanese and Taiwanese. The recipes are based on traditional food from these countries that are healthy without being bland or boring. These recipes are also vegan and gluten-free. Heartiest Dishes: These dishes are full of protein and carbohydrates as well as vitamins and minerals. The meals are hearty but leave you feeling full so you don't need to eat constantly. They feature a variety of meats, beans and vegetables. These dishes make great entrees or side dishes.

These dishes are full of protein and carbohydrates as well as vitamins and minerals. The meals are hearty but leave you feeling full so you don't need to eat constantly. They feature a variety of meats, beans and vegetables. These dishes make great entrees or side dishes. Energy Boosts: These dishes are tasty and nutritious but also relatively low in calories. They will provide the boost you need to recover from a hard workout or day at work.

Most people don't have time to cook healthy food, but that doesn't mean it's out of the question. On the contrary, people should always be trying to incorporate healthy eating into their lives. There are many ways for you to do this, such as making changes to your diet or stocking your pantry with nutritious ingredients. This will help you better control your diabetes and overall health.

21 Days Meal Plan

Day	Breakfast	Lunch	Dinner	Dessert
1	Basil Tomato Frittata	Almond Pancakes	Zucchini Salmon Salad	Spinach and Artichoke Dip
2	Coconut Bread	Mouth-watering Pie	Pan Fried Salmon	Buffalo Dip
3	Chia Spinach Pancakes	Peanut Butter and Cacao Breakfast Quinoa	Grilled Salmon with Pineapple Salsa	Potato Wedges
4	Olive Cheese Omelet	Chicken Omelet	Mediterranean Chickpea Salad	Dill Hummus
5	Feta Kale Frittata	Almond Coconut Cereal	Warm Chorizo Chickpea Salad	Latte Pudding
6	Fresh Berry Muffins	WW Salad in a Jar	Tomato Fish Bake	Peanut Butter
7	Cheese Zucchini Eggplant	Almond Porridge	Garlicky Tomato Chicken Casserole	Vegan Crackers
8	Broccoli Nuggets	Special Almond Cereal	Chicken Cacciatore	Spelt Banana Bread
9	Cauliflower Frittata	Bacon and Lemon spiced Muffins	Fennel Wild Rice Risotto	Yeast-Free Spelt Bread
10	Coconut Kale Muffins	Greek Style Mini Burger Pies	Wild Rice Prawn Salad	Flatbread

11	Protein Muffins	Awesome Avocado Muffins	Chicken Broccoli Salad with Avocado Dressing	Chickpea Loaf
12	Healthy Waffles	Raw-Cinnamon-Apple Nut Bowl	Seafood Paella	Zucchini Bread Pancakes
13	Cheese Almond Pancakes	Family Fun Pizza	Herbed Roasted Chicken Breasts	Kamut and Raisin Pancakes
14	Vegetable Quiche	Tasty WW Pancakes	Marinated Chicken Breasts	Spelt and Strawberry Waffles
15	Pumpkin Muffins	Slow Cooker Savory Butternut Squash Oatmeal	Greek Style Quesadillas	Chickpea and Quinoa Burgers
16	Pancakes with Berries	Yummy Smoked Salmon	Creamy Penne	Teff Burgers
17	Omelette À La Margherita	WW Breakfast Cereal	Light Paprika Moussaka	Chickpea Nuggets
18	Porridge with Walnuts	Avocados Stuffed with Salmon	Cucumber Bowl with Spices and Greek Yogurt	Pumpkin Spice Crackers
19	Alkaline Blueberry Spelt Pancakes	Green Lamb Curry	Stuffed Bell Peppers with Quinoa	Spicy Roasted Nuts
20	Ancho Tilapia on Cauliflower Rice	Lemon Lamb Chops	Mediterranean Burrito	Potato Chips

Breakfast Recipes

1. Fresh Berry Muffins

Difficulty: Average

Preparation Time: 11 minutes

Cooking Time: 26 minutes

Servings: 9

Ingredients:

- 2 eggs (1 lean)

- ½ tsp vanilla (1/4 condiment)

- 1/2 cup fresh blueberries (1/2 healthy fat)

- 1 tsp baking powder (1/8 condiment)

- 6 drops stevia (1/4 condiment)

- 1 cup heavy cream (1/2 healthy fat)

- 2 cups almond flour (1/4 condiment)

- 1/4 cup butter, melted (1/2 healthy fat)

Directions:

1. Set the oven to 350 F.

2. Stir in eggs to the mixing bowl and whisk until well mix.

3. Mix in remaining ingredients to the eggs.

4. Fill in the batter into a greased muffin tray and bake in the oven

for 25 minutes. Serve.

Nutrition:

190 Calories

18g Fat

5.4g Protein

2. Cheese Zucchini Eggplant

Difficulty: Easy

Preparation Time: 10 minutes Cooking Time: 2 hours

Servings: 8

Ingredients:

• 1 eggplant, cut in 1-inch cubes (1 green)

• 1 ½ cup spaghetti sauce (1 healthy fat)

• 1 medium zucchini, cut into 1-inch pieces (1 green)

• 1/2 cup parmesan cheese, shredded (1/2 healthy fat)

Directions:

1. Incorporate all ingredients into the crock pot and stir well.

2. Cover and cook on high for 2 hours.

3. Stir well and serve.

Nutrition:

47 Calories 1.2g Fat 2.5g Protein

3. Broccoli Nuggets

Difficulty: Easy

Preparation Time: 10 minutes

Cooking Time: 15 minutes

Servings: 4

Ingredients:

- 2 egg whites (1 lean)

- 2 cups broccoli florets (2 green)

- 1/4 cup almond flour (1/4 condiment)

- 1 cup cheddar cheese, shredded (1/2 condiment)

- 1/8 tsp salt (1/8 condiment)

Directions:

1. Preheat the oven to 350 F.

2. Add broccoli in bowl and mash using a masher.

3. Stir in remaining ingredients to the broccoli.

4. Place 20 scoops onto a baking tray and press lightly down.

5.   Bake in preheated oven for 20 minutes.

6.   Serve and enjoy.

Nutrition:

145 Calories

10.4g Fat

10.56g Protein

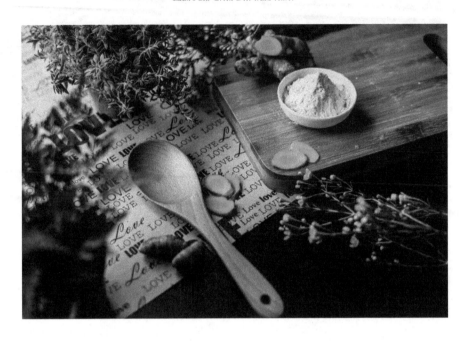

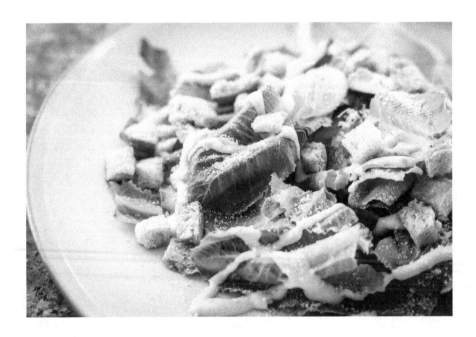

Lunch Recipes

4. Easy Keto Chicken Soup

Preparation Time: 10 minutes

Cooking Time: 1 hour

Servings: 14

Ingredients:

- 2 cups of Shredded chicken, cooked

- 1 cup of Carrots, diced

- 1 cup Celery, diced

- 1 cup of Onion, diced

- 10 cups of Chicken broth

- 1 tablespoon of Italian seasoning

- 1 Bay leaf

- A dash of Sea salt

- A dash of Black pepper

- 1 Spaghetti squash

Directions:

1.   Combine all the Ingredients: minus the spaghetti squash in a pot over medium heat. Cook until it boils, then decrease to a simmer and cover the pot. Cook for one hour.

2.   Next, preheat the oven to about 375 degrees F, then punch holes in the spaghetti squash with a knife. Transfer to a baking sheet and bake in the oven for sixty minutes.

3.   When the spaghetti squash is cooked, cut in half and scoop out the strands using a fork. Remove the bay leaf and add in half of the spaghetti squash strands.

Nutrition:

Calories: 44 Carbohydrates: 4g Protein: 5g

Fat: 1g

5. Taco Casserole

Preparation Time: 30 minutes

Cooking Time: 1 Hour

Servings: 8

Ingredients:

- 1 lb. Ground Turkey

- 1 Cauliflower, Small & Chopped into Florets

- 1 Jalapeno Diced

- ¼ Cup Red Peppers, Diced

- ¼ Cup Onion, Diced

- 1 Teaspoon Cumin

- 1 Teaspoon Parsley

- 1 Teaspoon Garlic Minced

- 1 Teaspoon Turmeric

- 1 Teaspoon Oregano

- 1 ½ Cups Cheddar Cheese, Shredded

- 1 Cup Sour Cream

Directions:

1.   Put your minced meat and cauliflower in a bowl before adding

all your herbs and spices. Stir in your red peppers, jalapenos and onions

together, mixing in a cup of your cheese.

2.   Pour into a casserole dish before topping with remaining cheese.

3.   Bake at 350 for an hour and serve with sour cream.

Nutrition:

Calories: 242 Protein: 18 Grams

Fat: 17 Grams

Net Carbs: 4 Grams

6. Quick Keto Roasted Tomato Soup

Preparation Time: 5 minutes Cooking Time: 40 minutes

Servings: 6

Ingredients:

- 10 fresh Rome tomato, sliced into tubes

- 2 tablespoons of Olive oil

- 4 cloves of Garlic, minced

- 2 cup of Chicken bone broth

- 1 tablespoon of Herbs de Provence

- 1/2 teaspoon of Sea salt

- 1/4 teaspoon of Black pepper

- 1/4 cup of Heavy cream

- 2 tablespoons of Fresh basil

Directions:

1. First, preheat the oven to about 400 degrees F, then line a baking sheet with some foil, then grease the foil.

2.   Mix the tomato chunks with minced garlic and olive oil. Place the tomato chunks on a baking sheet.

3.   Transfer to the oven and bake until the skin wrinkles, about twenty-five minutes.

4.   Remove from the heat and put the tomato chunks into the blender and blend until smooth.

5.   Pour the tomato puree into the pot and place over medium-high heat. Add in the broth and season with sea salt, herbs de Provence, and black pepper. Boil for about fifteen minutes.

6.   Add in the basil and cream and serve.

Nutrition:

Calories: 95

Fat: 8g

Protein: 3g

Carbohydrates: 3g

Dinner Recipes

7. Steak and Mushroom Noodles

Preparation time: 10 minutes

Cooking time: 20 minutes

Servings: 4

Ingredients:

- 100g shitake mushrooms, halved, if large

- 100g chestnut mushrooms, sliced

- 150g udon noodles

- 75g kale, finely chopped

- 75g baby leaf spinach, chopped

- 2 sirloin steaks

- 2 teaspoons miso paste

- 2.5cm piece fresh ginger, finely chopped

- 1 star anise

- 1 red chili, finely sliced

- 1 red onion, finely chopped

- 1 fresh coriander (cilantro) chopped

- 1 liter (1½ pints) warm water

Directions:

1.   Pour the water into a saucepan and add in the miso, star anise, and ginger. Bring it to the boil, reduce the heat, and simmer gently. In the meantime, cook the noodles according to their instructions, then drain them.

2.   Heat the oil in a saucepan, add the steak and cook for around 2-3 minutes on each side (or 1-2 minutes, for rare meat).

3.   Remove the meat and set aside.

4.   Place the mushrooms, spinach, coriander (cilantro), and kale into the miso broth and cook for 5 minutes.

5.   In the meantime, heat the remaining oil in a separate pan and fry the chili and onion for 4 minutes, until softened.

6.   Serve the noodles into bowls and pour the soup on top.

7.   Thinly slice the steaks and add them to the top. Serve immediately.

Nutrition:

Calories: 296

Carbs: 24

Fat: 13

Protein: 32

8. Masala Scallops

Preparation time: 10 minutes

Cooking time: 20 minutes

Servings: 4

Ingredients:

- 2 jalapenos, chopped

- 1 pound sea scallops

- A pinch of salt and black pepper

- ¼ teaspoon cinnamon powder

- 1 teaspoon garam masala

- 1 teaspoon coriander, ground

- 1 teaspoon cumin, ground

- 2 tablespoons cilantro, chopped

Directions:

1.   Heat up a pan with the oil over medium heat, add the jalapenos, cinnamon, and the other ingredients except for the scallops and cook for 10 minutes.

Nutrition:

Calories: 251

Fat: 4g

Carbs: 11g

Protein: 17g

9. Tuna and Tomatoes

Preparation time: 5 minutes

Cooking time: 20 minutes

Servings: 4

Ingredients:

- 1 yellow onion, chopped

- 1 tablespoon olive oil

- 1 cup tomatoes, chopped

- 1 red pepper, chopped • 1 teaspoon sweet paprika

- 1 tablespoon coriander, chopped

Directions:

1. Heat up a pan with the oil over medium heat, add the onions and the pepper and cook for 5 minutes.

2.	Add the fish and the other ingredients, cook everything for 15 minutes, divide between plates and serve.

Nutrition:

Calories: 215

Fat: 4g

Carbs: 14g

Protein: 7g

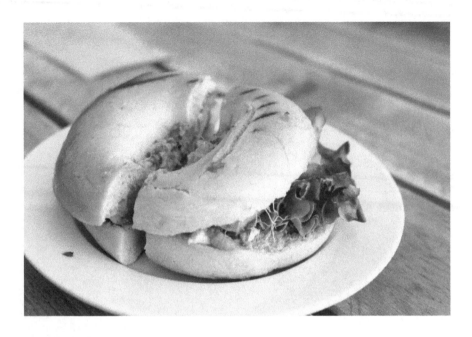

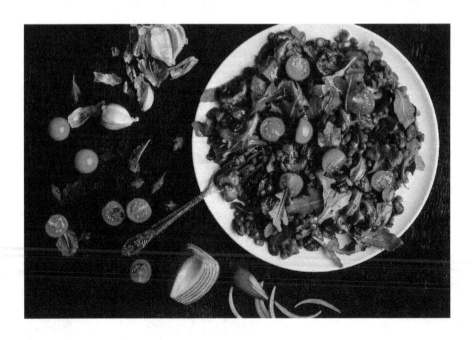

Meat Recipes

10. Pork Tenderloins and Mushrooms

Preparation Time: 10 minutes

Cooking Time: 25 minutes

Serve: 4

Ingredients:

- on-stick cooking spray 1 Tablespoon garlic

- 1 Tablespoon marjoram

- 1 Tablespoon basil

- 1 Tablespoon onion

- 1 Tablespoon parsley

- 1 1/2 lbs. pork tenderloin (or beef tenderloin, or chicken breasts) 6 cups portobello mushroom caps, cut into chunks

- 1/2 C low sodium chicken broth

- 1 Tablespoon Stacey Hawkins Garlic Gusto or Garlic & Spring

- Onion Seasoning (or garlic, salt, black pepper, onion, paprika, and parsley)

- fresh parsley for garnish if desired

Direction:

1.Spray a large skillet with cooking spray.

2.Preheat the stove to medium heat.

3.Place garlic and herbs into the skillet to cook with the cooking spray.

4.Allow the garlic and herbs to cook for 1 minute.

5.Place the pork tenderloin into the pan.

6.Generously season the pork tenderloin with the garlic gusto.

7.Sear the pork for 5 minutes and flip to the other side. Cook the other-

side for another 1 minute.

8.Add the mushrooms, broth, and 2 tablespoons of water into the pan.

9.Cover the pan for 20 minutes.

10.Uncover and simmer for an additional 10,5 minutes till tender.

11.Garnish with marjoram. Serve hot.

Nutrition:

Energy (calories): 737 kcal Protein: 30.32 g Fat: 62.95 g Carbohydrates:

14.39 g Calcium, Ca40 mg Magnesium, Mg48 mg Phosphorus, P443 mg

11. **Garlic Shrimp & Broccoli**

Preparation Time: 15 min and 30 min marinade

Cooking Time: 8 minutes

Serve: 4

Ingredients:

- 1/2 cup honey

- 1/4 cup soy sauce

- 1 teaspoon fresh grated ginger

- 2 tablespoons minced garlic

- 1/4 teaspoon red pepper flakes

- 1/2 teaspoon cornstarch

- 1-pound large shrimp, peeled, deveined, and tails removed if desired

- 2 tablespoon butter

- 2 cups chopped broccoli

- 1 teaspoon olive oil

- salt pepper

Direction:

1.In a large-bowl, combine honey, soy sauce, ginger, garlic, red pepper flakes, and cornstarch. Add shrimp and toss to combine. Cover and refrigerate for 23 to 33 minutes.

2.Stir-fry in a cast iron pan:

3.In a big-nonstick skillet, heat 1 normal spoon of the butter and olive oil over medium-high heat. Cook and stir broccoli in the hot skillet until crisp-tender, occasionally stirring, 2 to 4 minutes. Remove broccoli from skillet.

4.Add shrimp mixture to hot skillet and stir-fry for 4-5 minutes or until

shrimp are done. Stir in broccoli and add salt and pepper to taste.

5.Remove from the heat.

6.Serve with rice; your family will love it!

Nutrition: Energy (calories):

334 kcal Protein: 17.84 g Fat: 11.07 g Carbohydrates: 43.4 g Calcium,

Ca100 mg Magnesium, Mg42 mg Phosphorus, P324 mg

12. Chicken with Garlic and Spring Onion Cream

Preparation Time: 5 minutes Cooking Time: 15 minutes Serve: 4

Ingredients:

•   6 medium chicken breasts

•   3 spoons butter or 3 spoons margarine 2 spoons all-purpose flour • One-third cup chopped green onion Three-fourth cup chicken broth One-fourth teaspoon salt

•   pepper •   1 -2 tablespoon Dijon mustard (to taste) 1 cup plain yogurt

Direction:

1.Heat a large skillet, add 1 tablespoon butter. Add chicken breasts to the pan. Cook for 10 minutes on medium heat, until browned on both sides. Remove and set aside on a plate.

2.Flour a chopping board and cut chicken breasts into thin strips when you're free from extra fat.

3.Melt 2 spoons butter in the same skillet. Stir in flour and cook for 2 minutes, stirring constantly. Gradually add chicken broth, mustard, salt, and pepper. (For a thicker sauce, add 2 tablespoons cornstarch dissolved in 1/2 cup cold water.)

4.Blend in yogurt. Add chicken strips and green onion. Cook until sauce bubbles and thickens, stirring occasionally.

5.Serve with plain white rice or boiled potatoes.

Nutrition:

Energy (calories): 1172 kcal Protein: 132.83 g Fat: 63.49 g Carbohydrates: 9.7 g Calcium, Ca162 mg Magnesium, Mg155 mg Phosphorus, P1073 mg

13. Pan-Seared Beef Tips and Mushrooms

Preparation Time: 10 minutes Cooking Time: 25 minutes

Serve: 4

Ingredients:

- 1 1/2 lbs. lean beef cut into 1 chunk (London broil, filet, strip steak, etc.)

- 1/2 T salt 1/2 T pepper 1/2 T garlic

- nonstick cooking spray

- 4 C mushrooms (either small, whole mushrooms or larger ones cut into quarters)

- 1 C low sodium beef broth 11/2 teaspoons fresh garlic 11/2 teaspoons parsley 11/2 teaspoons onion

Direction:

1.Sprinkle beef with salt, pepper, and garlic.

2.Coat large skillet with nonstick cooking spray. Heat over medium-high heat and add beef. Cook about 8-10 minutes, stirring frequently or until beef is browned on all sides and no pink remains.

3.Add mushrooms to the skillet. Pour beef broth and boil. Cover and cook over low-heat for 15 minutes.

4.While beef simmers in mushroom sauce, combine garlic, parsley, and onion in a food processor fitted with a steel blade. Pulse a few times until minced.

5.Add garlic mixture to beef and mushrooms and simmer covered for 10 minutes more. 6.Place in the serving bowl and season with parsley. As an alternative, if desired, top with gouda cheese.

Nutrition:

Energy (calories): 379 kcal Protein: 42.49 g Fat: 12.44 g Carbohydrates: 25.55 g Calcium, Ca66 mg Magnesium, Mg69 mg

14. Creamy Skillet Chicken and Asparagus

Preparation Time: 5 minutes

Cooking Time: 20 minutes

Serve: 4

Ingredients:

• 1 1/2 tablespoon extra-virgin olive oil

• Salt and fresh-ground pepper to taste, 4 (1 pound) boneless skinless chicken breasts

• 2 spoons Italian Seasoning 1 tablespoon butter

• 1-pound asparagus stalks trimmed and cut into thirds 1 yellow onion sliced

• 1 cup fat-free half & half 1/2 tablespoon all-purpose 1/3 cup grated Parmesan flour

• Lemon slices of salt and fresh ground pepper to taste for garnishing chopped parsley for garnishing freshly rubbed parmesan to garnish

Direction:

1.Heat a big nonstick omelet pans over medium-high heat. Add olive oil and swirl. Season chicken with salt and pepper and Italian season. Add chicken to the pan and sauté until the tops are brown, about 4 minutes, then flip and cook another 4,3-5,3 minutes, or until golden.

2.Remove chicken from pan and keep warm. Add butter to the pan, asparagus, onion, and sauté until the asparagus is tender, about 4 mins.

3.Season the asparagus. Sprinkle in the flour, constantly stirring, until the mixture is homogenized and bubbly. Gradually add the 1/2 cup of half and half, constantly stirring, then add parmesan cheese, garlic, lemon juice, salt, and pepper.

4.Cook until sauce thickens, about 2 minutes. Taste and adjust seasoning. Stir in the rest of the half and half. Add chicken back into the pan to reheat and toss together with the sauce.

5.Remove from heat and onto the plates. Serve and garnish with lemon-slices, parsley, and parmesan.

Nutrition:

Energy (calories): 703 kcal Protein: 110.07 g Fat: 18.54 g Carbohydrates: 19.52 g Calcium, Ca190 mg Magnesium, Mg171 mg

15. Rump Steak

Preparation Time: 15 Minutes

Cooking Time: 10 Minutes

Servings: 3

Ingredients

1 pound of rump steak

1 onion, sliced

1 green bell pepper, sliced

Salt and black pepper, to taste

1 cup parmesan cheese

Hoagies roll, as needed

Directions

1.   Add steak, bell pepper, and onion in an air fryer basket.

2.   Season it with salt and black pepper.

3.   Place it inside air fryer.

4.   Let it Bake for 8 minutes at 350 degrees F.

5.   Once done, place it on a hoagie roll.

6.   Sprinkle it with parmesan cheese.

7.   Serve.

Serving Suggestion: Serve with Mashed Potatoes

Variation Tip: Use mozzarella cheese Instead of parmesan

Nutritional Information per Serving:

Calories 391| Fat 25g| Sodium 1000mg | Carbs 0.4g| Fiber 0.1g |

Sugar 0.1g | Protein 42g

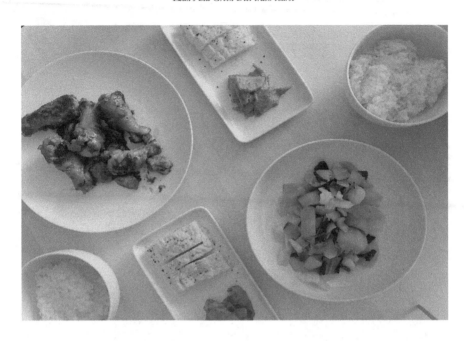

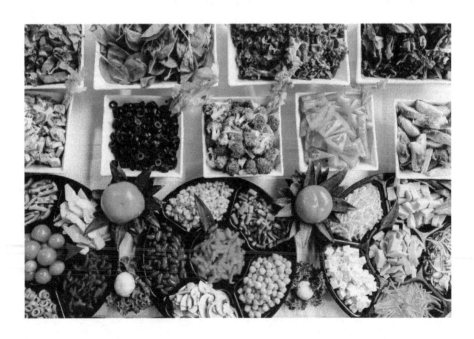

Poultry Recipes

16. Turkey Pepper Kabobs

Preparation time: 15 minutes

Marinating Grill: 10 minutes

Servings: 4

Ingredients:

Eight-ounces unsweetened pineapple chunks

1/4 cup brown sugar

Two tablespoons canola oil

Two tablespoons Worcestershire sauce

One garlic clove – minced

One teaspoon prepared mustard

One pound turkey breast tenderloins – cut into 1-inch cubes

One sweet onion – cut into 3/4-inch pieces

One green pepper – cut into one-inch pieces

One sweet red pepper – cut into one-inch pieces

Direction:

Drain pineapple and reserve ¼ cup juice.

1. For the marinade: combine reserved juice, garlic, mustard, oil, brown sugar, and Worcestershire sauce.

2. Toss turkey with 1/3 cup marinade in another bowl. Place into the fridge and cover with a lid for two hours.

3. Cover the remaining marinade and place it into the fridge.

4. Thread pineapple chunks, vegetables, and turkey on the soaked wooden skewers.

5. Place kabobs on the oiled grill and heat over medium flame.

6. Cook for eight to ten minutes. Baste with reserved marinade during the last three minutes and serve!

Nutrition:

Calories 298 | fat 6g | sodium 146mg | carbohydrate 34g | fiber 3g | sugar 28g | protein 30g

17. Asparagus Turkey Stir-Fry

Preparation time: 20 minutes

Servings: 4

Ingredients:

Two teaspoons cornstarch

1/4 cup chicken broth

One tablespoon lemon juice

One teaspoon soy sauce

One pound turkey breast tenderloins – cut into half-inch strips

One garlic clove – minced

Two tablespoons canola oil

One-pound fresh asparagus – trimmed and cut into 1-1/2-inch pieces

- Two-ounces sliced pimientos – drained

Direction:

1. Mix the soy sauce, lemon juice, broth, and cornstarch into the bowl and keep it aside.

2. Add turkey and garlic in one tablespoon oil into the wok and cook until no longer pink.

3. Add asparagus in oil and cook until tender.

4. Add pimientos and broth mixture to the pan. Cook for one minute until thick.

5. Place turkey back to the pan and cook well.

6. Serve!

Nutrition:

Calories 205 | fat 9g | sodium 204mg | carbohydrate 5g | fiber 1g | sugar 1g | protein 28g

18. Peanut Turkey Satay

Preparation time: 15 minutes Servings: 2

Ingredients:

4-1/2 teaspoons red wine vinegar

4-1/2 teaspoons reduced-sodium soy sauce

One tablespoon sugar

One tablespoon creamy peanut butter

1/4 teaspoon ground ginger

Half pound turkey breast tenderloins

Direction:

1. Add red wine vinegar, soy sauce, sugar, creamy peanut butter, and ground ginger into the bowl. Keep it aside. Reserve one tablespoon for basting.

2. Cut turkey into long strips. Add to soy sauce mixture and toss well until combine.

3. Thread turkey strips onto two soaked wooden skewers.

4. Broil for two to three minutes.

5. Baste with reserved soy sauce mixture.

Nutrition:

Calories 202 | fat 6g | sodium 552mg | carbohydrate 9g | fiber 1g | sugar 7g | protein 29g

19. Spinach-Pesto Turkey Tenderloins

Preparation time: 20 minutes

Baking time: 25 minutes

Serving: 4

Ingredients:

Six cups fresh baby spinach - 6 ounces, chopped

One cup crumbled goat cheese

Two garlic cloves – minced

Two turkey breast tenderloins – 8 ounces each

1/3 cup prepared pesto

1/4 cup shredded Parmesan cheese

Direction:

1. Preheat the oven to 350 degrees Fahrenheit.

2. Add water into the saucepan and boil it. Add spinach and boil for three to five minutes, and drain well.

3. Mix the garlic, cheese, and spinach into the bowl.

4. Slice tenderloin horizontally and fill with cheese mixture.

5. Secure with kitchen strings.

6. Next, place tenderloin on the greased baking pan and brush with pesto.

7. Place into the oven and bake for five to ten minutes.

8. Cut tenderloin into four pieces.

Nutrition:

Calories 306 | fat 19g | sodium 458mg | carbohydrate 5g | fiber 3g | sugar 0 | protein 32g.

20. Butter Chicken

Preparation time: 15 minutes

Cooking time: 28 minutes

Servings: 5

Ingredients:

- 3 tablespoons unsalted butter

- 1 medium yellow onion, chopped

- 2 garlic cloves, minced

- 1 teaspoon fresh ginger, minced

- 1½ pounds grass-fed chicken breasts, cut into ¾-inch chunks

- 2 tomatoes, chopped finely

- 1 tablespoon garam masala

- 1 teaspoon red chili powder

- 1 teaspoon ground cumin

- Salt and ground black pepper, as required

- 1 cup heavy cream

- 2 tablespoons fresh cilantro, chopped

Directions:

1. Melt butter in a large wok over medium-high heat and sauté the onions for about 5–6 minutes.

2. Now, add in ginger and garlic and sauté for about 1 minute.

3. Add the tomatoes and cook for about 2–3 minutes, crushing with the back of the spoon.

4. Stir in the chicken spices, salt, and black pepper, and cook for about 6–8 minutes or until the desired doneness of the chicken.

5. Stir in the heavy cream and cook for about 8–10 more minutes, stirring occasionally.

6.   Garnish with fresh cilantro and serve hot.

Nutrition: Calories 506, Fat 22, Carbs 4, Protein 32

21. Baked Chicken Fajitas

Preparation time: 10 minutes

Cooking time: 18 minutes

Servings: 6

Ingredients:

- 1 1/2 lbs. chicken tenders

- 2 tbsp fajita seasoning

- 2 tbsp olive oil

- 1 onion, sliced

- 2 bell pepper, sliced

- 1 lime juice • 1 tsp kosher salt

Directions:

1. Preheat the oven to 400 F.

2.   Add all ingredients in a large mixing bowl and toss well.

3.   Transfer bowl mixture on a baking tray and bake in preheated

oven for 15-18 minutes.

4.   Serve and enjoy.

Nutrition: Calories 286, Fat 13, Carbs 7, Protein 33

Fish and Seafood Recipes

22. Arugula and Sweet Potato Salad

Preparation Time: 10 Minutes

Cooking Time: 20 Minutes

Servings: 4

Ingredients:

- 1 lb. Sweet potatoes

- 1 Cup walnuts

- 1 Tablespoon olive oil

- 1 Cup water

- 1 Tablespoon soy sauce

- 3 Cups arugula

Directions:

1.   Bake potatoes at 400°F until tender, remove, and set aside.

2.   In a bowl, drizzle walnuts with olive oil and microwave for 2-3 minutes or until toasted.

3.   In a bowl, combine all salad ingredients and mix well.

4.   Pour over the soy sauce and serve.

Nutrition:

Calories: 189

Total Carbohydrate: 2g

Cholesterol: 13mg Total Fat: 7g Fiber: 2g

Protein: 10g

Sodium: 301mg

23. Black Cod

Preparation Time: 15 Minutes

Cooking Time: 20 Minutes

Servings: 4

Ingredients:

- ¼ Cup miso paste

- ¼ Cup's sake

- 1 Tablespoon mirin

- 1 Teaspoon soy sauce

- 1 Tablespoon olive oil

- 4 Black cod filets

Directions:

1.   In a bowl, combine miso, soy sauce, oil, and sake.

2.   Rub mixture over cod fillets and let it marinate for 20-30 minutes.

3.   Adjust broiler and broil cod filets for 10-12 minutes.

4.   Remove and serve when the fish is done.

Nutrition:

Calories: 231

Total Carbohydrate: 2g

Cholesterol: 13mg

Total Fat: 15g

Fiber: 2g

Protein: 8g

Sodium: 298mg

24. Buttery Cod

Preparation Time: 10 Minutes

Cooking Time: 12 Minutes

Servings: 2

Ingredients:

- 2 x 4-oz. Cod fillets

- 2 Tbsp. salted butter, melted

- 1 Tsp. Old Bay seasoning

- ½ Medium lemon, sliced

Directions:

1.   Place the cod fillets in a skillet.

2.   Brush with melted butter, season with Old Bay, and top with a few lemon wedges.

3.   Wrap the fish in aluminum foil and place it in your deep fryer.

4.   Cook for eight minutes at 350°F.

5.   The cod is done when it is easily peeled. Serve hot.

Nutrition:

Calories: 394

Fat: 5g

Protein: 12g

Sugar: 4g

25. Salmon Pasta

Preparation Time: 10 Minutes

Cooking Time: 25 Minutes

Servings: 2

Ingredients:

- 5 Tablespoons butter

- ¼ Onion

- 1 Tablespoon all-purpose flour

- 1 Teaspoon garlic powder

- 2 Cups skim milk

- ¼ Cup Romano cheese

- 1 Cup green peas

- ¼ Cup canned mushrooms

- 8 oz. Salmon

- 1 Package penne pasta

Directions:

1.   Bring a pot with water to a boil.

2.   Add pasta and cook for 10-12 minutes.

3.   In a skillet, melt butter, add onion, and sauté until tender.

4.   Stir in garlic powder, flour, milk, and cheese.

5.   Add mushrooms, peas and cook on low heat for 4-5 minutes.

6.   Toss in salmon and cook for another 2-3 minutes.

7.   When ready, serve with cooked pasta.

Nutrition:

Calories: 211 Total Carbohydrate: 7g Cholesterol: 13mg

Total Fat: 18g Fiber: 3g Protein: 17g Sodium: 289mg

26. Bass Filet in Coconut Sauce

Preparation Time: 5 minutes

Cooking Time: 15 minutes

Servings: 4

Ingredients:

- ¼ cup coconut milk • ½ pound bass fillet

- 1 tablespoon olive oil

- 2 tablespoons jalapeno, chopped

- 2 tablespoons lime juice, freshly squeezed

- 3 tablespoons parsley, chopped

- Salt and pepper to taste

Directions:

1. Preheat the air fryer for 5 minutes

2.   Season the bass with salt and pepper to taste

3.   Brush the surface with olive oil.

4.   Put in the air fryer and cook for 15 minutes at 3500F.

5.   Meanwhile, place in a saucepan, the coconut milk, lime juice, jalapeno and parsley.

6.   Heat over medium flame.

7.   Serve the fish with the coconut sauce.

Nutrition:

Calories 139

Carbohydrates: 2.7g

Protein: 8.7g

Fat: 10.3

Side Dish Recipes

27. Salty Lemon Artichokes

Preparation Time: 15 minutes   Cooking Time: 45 minutes

Servings: 2

Ingredients:

- 1 lemon

- 2 artichokes

- 1 teaspoon kosher salt

- 1 garlic head

- 2 teaspoons olive oil

Directions:

1. Cut off the edges of the artichokes.

2.   Cut the lemon into the halves.

3.   Peel the garlic head and chop the garlic cloves roughly.

4.   Then place the chopped garlic in the artichokes.

5.   Sprinkle the artichokes with the olive oil and kosher salt.

6.   Then squeeze the lemon juice into the artichokes.

7.   Wrap the artichokes in the foil.

8.   Preheat the air fryer to 330 F.

9.   Place the wrapped artichokes in the air fryer and cook for 45 minutes.

10.   When the artichokes are cooked – discard the foil and serve.

11.   Enjoy!

Nutrition: Calories: 133 Fat: 5g Fiber: 9.7g Carbs: 21.7g Protein: 6g

28. Asparagus & Parmesan

Preparation Time: 10 minutes

Cooking Time: 6 minutes

Servings: 2

Ingredients:

- 1 teaspoon sesame oil

- 11 oz. asparagus

- 1 teaspoon chicken stock

- ½ teaspoon ground white pepper

- 3 oz. Parmesan

Directions:

1.   Wash the asparagus and chop it roughly.

2.   Sprinkle the chopped asparagus with the chicken stock and ground white pepper.

3.   Then sprinkle the vegetables with the sesame oil and shake them. 4.   Place the asparagus in the air fryer basket.

5.   the vegetables for 4 minutes at 400 F.

6.   Meanwhile, shred Parmesan cheese.

7.   When the time is over – shake the asparagus gently and sprinkle with the shredded cheese.

8.   Cook the asparagus for 2 minutes more at 400 F.

9.   After this, transfer the cooked asparagus in the serving plates.

10.   Serve and taste it!

Nutrition: Calories: 189 Fat: 11.6g Fiber: 3.4g Carbs: 7.9g Protein: 17.2g

Soup and Salad Recipes

29. Minestrone Soup

Preparation Time: 10 minutes

Cooking Time: 25 minutes

Servings: 4 servings

Ingredients:

• 1 ½ cup ground pork

• ½ bell pepper, chopped

• 2 tablespoons chives, chopped

• 2 oz. celery stalk, chopped

• 1 teaspoon butter

• 1 teaspoon Italian seasonings

• 4 cups chicken broth • ½ cup mushrooms, sliced

Directions:

1. Heat up butter on the sauté mode for 2 minutes.

2. Add bell pepper. Cook the vegetable for 5 minutes.

3. Then stir them well and add mushrooms, celery stalk, and Italian seasonings. Stir well and cook for 5 minutes more.

4. Add ground pork, chives, and chicken broth.

5. Close and seal the lid.

6. Cook the soup on manual mode (high pressure) for 15 minutes. Make a quick pressure release.

Nutrition:

Calories 408 Fat 27.2 Fiber 0.6 Carbs 3 Protein 35.6

30. Chorizo Soup

Preparation Time: 10 minutes

Cooking Time: 17 minutes

Servings: 3 servings

Ingredients:

• 8 oz. chorizo, chopped

• 1 teaspoon tomato paste

• 4 oz. scallions, diced

• 1 tablespoon dried cilantro

• ½ teaspoon chili powder

• 1 teaspoon avocado oil • 2 cups beef broth

Directions:

1. Heat up avocado oil on sauté mode for 1 minute.

2. Add chorizo and cook it for 6 minutes, stir it from time to time.

3. Then add scallions, tomato paste, cilantro, and chili powder. Stir well.

4. Add beef broth.

5. Close and seal the lid.

6. Cook the soup on manual mode (high pressure) for 10 minutes. Make a quick pressure release.

Nutrition:

Calories 387

Fat 30.2

Fiber 1.3

Carbs 5.5

Protein 22.3

31. Red Feta Soup

Preparation Time: 10 minutes

Cooking Time: 25 minutes

Servings: 4 servings

Ingredients:

• 1 cup broccoli, chopped

• 1 teaspoon tomato paste

• ½ cup coconut cream

• 4 cups beef broth

• 1 teaspoon chili flakes • 6 oz. feta, crumbled

Directions:

1. Put broccoli, tomato paste, coconut cream, and beef broth in the instant pot.

2. Add chili flakes and stir the mixture until it is red.

3. Then close and seal the lid and cook the soup for 8 minutes on manual mode (high pressure).

4. Then make a quick pressure release and open the lid.

5. Add feta cheese and sauté the soup on sauté mode for 5 minutes more.

Nutrition:

Calories 229

Fat 17.7

Fiber 1.3

Carbs 6.1

Protein 12.3

32. "Ramen" Soup

Preparation Time: 10 minutes

Cooking Time: 15 minutes

Servings: 2 servings

Ingredients:

• 1 zucchini, trimmed

• 2 cups chicken broth

• 2 eggs, boiled, peeled

• 1 tablespoon coconut amines

• 5 oz. beef loin, strips

• 1 teaspoon chili flakes

• 1 tablespoon chives, chopped

• ½ teaspoon salt

Directions:

1. Put the beef loin strips in the instant pot.

2. Add chili flakes, salt, and chicken broth.

3. Close and seal the lid. Cook the Ingredients: on manual mode (high pressure) for 15 minutes. Make a quick pressure release and open the lid.

4. Then make the s from zucchini with the help of the spiralizer and add them in the soup.

5. Add chives and coconut aminos.

6. Then ladle the soup in the bowls and top with halved eggs.

Nutrition:

Calories 254 Fat 11.8 Fiber 1.1 Carbs 6.2

Protein 30.6

33. Pepper Stuffing Soup

Preparation Time: 10 minutes

Cooking Time: 14 minutes

Servings: 4 servings

Ingredients:

• 1 cup ground beef

• ½ cup cauliflower, shredded

• 1 teaspoon dried oregano

• ½ teaspoon salt

• 1 teaspoon tomato paste

• 1 teaspoon minced garlic

• 4 cups of water

• ¼ cup of coconut milk

Directions:

1. Put all Ingredients in the instant pot bowl and stir well.

2. Then close and seal the lid.

3. Cook the soup on manual mode (high pressure) for 14 minutes.

4. When the time of cooking is finished, make a quick pressure release and open the lid.

Nutrition:

Calories 106

Fat 7.7

Fiber 0.9

Carbs 2.2

Protein 7.3

r

Lean and Green Recipe

34. Hearty Fruit Salad

Preparation time: 25 minutes

Cooking time: 5 minutes

Additional time: 3 hours

Servings: 10

Ingredients:

2/3 cup fresh orange juice

1/3 fresh lemon juice

1/3 cup packed brown sugar

Half teaspoon grated orange zest

Half teaspoon grated lemon zest

One teaspoon vanilla extract

Two cups cubed fresh pineapple

Two cups' strawberries – hulled and sliced

Three kiwi fruit – peeled and sliced

Three bananas – sliced

oranges – peeled and sectioned

One cup seedless grape

Two cups' blueberries

Direction:

1. Add lemon zest, orange, zest, brown sugar, lemon juice, and orange juice into the saucepan and boil over medium-high flame.

2. Decrease the speed of the flame to medium-low flame and simmer for five minutes.

3. Remove from the flame and add in vanilla extract.

4. Keep it aside to cool.

5. Next, layer the fruit in the glass bowl – pineapple, blueberries, grapes, oranges, bananas, kiwi fruits, and strawberries.

6. Add sauce over the fruit and cover with a lid. Place into the refrigerator for three to four hours.

Nutrition:

Calories 155 | fat 0.6g | sodium 4.7mg | carbohydrates 39g | fiber 4.5g | sugar 28.7g

| protein 1.8g

35. Vegan Waffles with Kale

Preparation time: 5 minutes

Cooking time: 10 minutes

Servings: 2

Ingredients:

For the Kale Mixture:

1.5 cups almond milk

One cup kale – stems removed

Half teaspoon pink salt

Three drop vanilla essence

Two teaspoon apple cider vinegar

Two tablespoon extra-virgin olive oil

1/4 cup fresh raspberries

One tablespoon brown sugar or coconut palm sugar

For the Batter:

1 1/4 cup all-purpose flour

Two teaspoon baking soda

1/4 cup almond milk

Direction:

1. Preheat the waffle iron.

2. Add all ingredients for the kale mixture into the blender.

3. Blend on low speed until combined well.

4. Put a sieve over the glass bowl and then add all-purpose flour and baking powder. Sieve it.

5. When sieved, add kale mixture.

6. Whisk the batter until no lumps remain.

7. If the batter is thick, add the extra almond milk.

8. Brush the waffle iron with vegan butter.

9. Add batter to the waffle iron and cook for eight to ten minutes.

10. Serve!

11. Top with maple syrup and fresh fruits.

12. You can add apple sauce, nutritional yeast, banana, chia seeds, hemp seeds, and flaxseed meal.

Nutrition:

Calories 487 | Fat 17g | Sodium 2140mg | Carbohydrates 71g | Fiber 3g | Sugar 6g | Protein 10g

36. Best Chia Pudding

Preparation Time: 10 minutes

Serving: 1

Ingredients:

3–4 tablespoons chia seeds

One cup milk

Half tablespoon maple syrup or honey

1/teaspoon vanilla

Toppings of choice: fresh berries or other fruit, granola, nut butter, etc.

Direction:

1. Add vanilla, maple syrup, milk, chia seeds into the bowl or Mason jar.

2. Place the lid and shake the mixture well.

3. When mixed, let rest for five minutes.

4. Shake well and cover with a lid. Place the mixture into the refrigerator for one to two hours.

5. Add more chia seeds and stir well and place into the refrigerator for a half-hour.

6. Top with berries.

7. Place into the air-tight container and put into the refrigerator for five to seven days.

Nutrition:

Calories 271 | Fat 16g | Sodium 248mg | Carbohydrates 26g | Fiber 16g | Sugar 6g | Protein 10g

Vegetables and Sides Recipes

37. Colorful Tabbouleh Salad

Preparation time: 15 minutes

Cooking time: 0 minutes

Servings: 4

Level of difficulty: Normal

Ingredients:

- 1 cup instant couscous

- salt and pepper to taste

- 4 tbsp. olive oil

- 2 1/2 tbsp. tomato paste

- 2 small tomato

- 7 sun-dried tomatoes in oil

- 2 spring onions

- 1 bunch parsley, fresh

- ½ cucumber

- 1 carrot

- 1 lemon (juiced)

- 1 1/2 cups vegetable broth (or just use water)

Optional

- 1 tbsp. Tabasco (or similar chili sauce)

- 2 tbsp. pumpkin seeds (or roasted sunflower seeds, to use as garnish)

- ½ bunch mint, fresh

Directions:

1.   Using vegetable broth for the tastiest results, cook the couscous according to packet instructions. Now add hot vegetable broth to it until it is all filled with the couscous.

2.   Position a tea-towel over the end. Give it a slight swirl after 3-4 minutes to make it fluffy. For 1 more minute, cover again.

3.   Rub the carrots and dice the cucumber, peppers, tomatoes (fresh and sun-dried), mint, and parsley in the meantime.

4.   With the cooked couscous, add the lemon juice, tomato paste, olive oil, salt, pepper, Tabasco sauce, and chopped and grated vegetables and herbs. Mix and serve. If using, garnish with seeds.

Nutrition:

Calories: 80| Carbs: 6g| Fat: 5g Protein: 1g

38. Easy Cauliflower Curry

Preparation time: 10 minutes

Cooking time: 20 minutes

Servings: 4

Level of difficulty: Normal

Ingredients:

- 1 bunch cilantro/coriander, fresh

- 1 tbsp. maple syrup • 1 tbsp. curry powder

- 1 lime (juiced)

- 1 can of coconut milk

- ½ tbsp. curry paste

- 1 tbsp. olive oil

- 2 thumbs ginger, fresh • 1 cup green beans

- 1 small-medium potato • ½ red peppers

- onions • Salt

- ½ medium cauliflowers

Directions:

1. Cut the cauliflower into bite-sized bits; slice the potatoes and bell pepper into small pieces. The tips of the green beans are separated and sliced in two.

2. Dice the onion and slice the ginger finely. Add some oil to a pan and add the ginger over medium heat.

3. Add the onion and bell pepper as soon as it begins to release its scent (about 2 minutes) and sauté (fry over medium heat) for 5 minutes. Mix in the paste of the curry, stir and simmer for another 2 minutes.

4. To dissolve the curry paste, stir in a little coconut milk and then add the remainder. Set to high heat before the milk begins to boil.

5.   Reduce to low heat and apply lime juice, curry powder, salt, and maple syrup until boiling. Only mix well.

6.   Now it is time for the potatoes and cauliflower to be added. Simmer for 5 minutes, add the green beans and leave to simmer for another 5 minutes.

7.   Give a taste test to the curry: see if you need any more salt, sugar, or lime to apply. You can even add a little more curry paste as well. It's ready to serve until you're comfortable.

8.   Serve on top of sliced new cilantro. With this lovely curry meal, rice or quinoa goes well!

Nutrition:

Calories: 475| Carbs: 45g| Fat: 24g| Protein: 26g

39. Spinach and Artichokes Sauté

Preparation Time: 20 minutes

Cooking Time: 15 minutes

Servings: 4

Ingredients:

• 10 oz. artichoke hearts, halved

• 2 cups baby spinach

• 3 garlic cloves

• ¼ cup veggie stock • 2 tsp. lime juice

• Salt and black pepper to taste

Directions:

1. In a pan that fits your air fryer, mix all the ingredients, toss, introduce

in the fryer, and cook at 370°F

for 15 minutes.

2. Divide between plates and serve as a side dish.

Nutrition:

Calories: 209 | Fats: 6 g| Carbs: 4 g| Protein: 8 g

40. Green Bean Casserole

Preparation Time: 25 minutes Cooking Time: 20 minutes

Servings: 4

Ingredients:

• 1 lb. fresh green beans, edges trimmed

• ½ oz. pork rinds, finely ground

• 1 oz. full -fat cream cheese

• ½ cup heavy whipping cream • ¼ cup diced yelp ow onion

• ½ cup chopped white mushrooms

• ½ cup chicken broth

• 4 tbsp. unsalted butter • ¼ tsp. xanthan gum

Directions:

1. Over heat, melt the butter in a skillet.

2. Sauté the onion and mushrooms until soft and fragrant, about 3-5 minutes.

3. Add the heavy cream, cream cheese, and broth to the skillet. Lightly beat until smooth. Boil and then simmer. Put the xanthan gum in the pan and remove from heat.

4. Cut green beans into 2-inch pieces and place in 4-cup round pan. Pour sauce mixture over them and stir until covered. Fil the plate with ground pork rinds. Place in the fryer basket.

5. Set the temperature to 320°F and set the timer for 15 minutes. The top will be a golden and green bean fork when fully cooked. Serve hot.

Nutrition:

Calories: 267| Fats: 23.4 g| Carbs: 9.7 g| Protein: 3.6 g

41. Black Bean Soup

Preparation Time: 10 minutes

Cooking Time: 20 minutes

Serving Size: 8 servings

Ingredients:

- tablespoons avocado oil

- 1 large onion, roughly chopped

- tablespoons garlic, minced

- 1 teaspoon ground cumin

- 15-oz cans of black beans, drained and rinsed

- 1½ cups corn

- 1 28-oz can dice tomatoes

- 1-quart vegetable stock

- teaspoons cayenne pepper (optional)

- sea salt and pepper to preference

Directions:

1. In a large soup pot, add olive oil, onion, and garlic. Cook over medium heat for 4 minutes.

2. Add beans, corn, tomatoes, and vegetable stock. Boil and then reduce heat to medium-low.

3. Add seasonings.

4. Simmer on low for 15 minutes and serve with your favorite toppings.

Nutritional Information Per Serving: 305 Calories, 7 grams of fat, 43 grams of Carbs, 10 grams of Protein

42. Jackfruit Vegetable Fry

Preparation Time: 5 minutes

Cooking Time: 5 minutes

Servings: 6

Ingredients:

- Two finely chopped small onions

- 2 cups finely chopped cherry tomatoes

- 1/8 tsp. ground turmeric

- 1 tbsp. olive oil

- Two seeded and chopped red bell peppers

- Three cups seeded and chopped firm jackfruit 1/8 tsp. cayenne

pepper

- 2 tbsps. chopped fresh basil leaves

- Salt

Directions:

1. In a greased skillet, sauté the onions and bell peppers for about 5 minutes.

2. Add the tomatoes, then stir.

3. Cook for 2 minutes.

4. Then add the jackfruit, cayenne pepper, salt, and turmeric.

5. Cook for about 8 minutes.

6. Garnish the meal with basil leaves.

7. Serve warm.

Nutrition: Calories: 236 kcal Fat: 1.8g Carbs: 48.3g Protein: 7g

Snacks and Dessert Recipes

43. Squash Salsa

Preparation time: 10 minutes

Cooking time: 3 hours

Servings: 2

Ingredients:

• 1 cup butternut squash, peeled and cubed

• 1 cup cherry tomatoes, cubed

• 1 cup avocado, peeled, pitted, and cubed

• ½ tablespoon balsamic vinegar

• ½ tablespoon lemon juice

• 1 tablespoon lemon zest, grated

• ¼ cup veggie stock

• 1 tablespoon chives, chopped

- A pinch of rosemary, dried

- A pinch of sage, dried

- A pinch of salt and black pepper

Directions:

1. In your slow cooker, mix the squash with the tomatoes, avocado, and the other ingredients, toss, put the lid on and cook on Low for 3 hours.

2. Divide into bowls and serve as a snack.

Nutrition:

calories 3886, fat 6, carbs 4, protein 12

44. Flavory Beans Spread

Preparation time: 10 minutes Cooking time: 6 hours Servings: 2

Ingredients:

- 1 cup canned black beans, drained

- 2 tablespoons tahini paste

- ½ teaspoon balsamic vinegar

- ¼ cup veggie stock

- ½ tablespoon olive oil

Directions:

1. In your slow cooker, mix the beans with the tahini paste and the other ingredients, toss, put the lid on and cook on Low for 6 hours.

2. Transfer to your food processor, blend well, divide into bowls, and serve.

Nutrition:

calories 432, fat 12, carbs 6, protein 4

45. Rice Bowls

Preparation time: 10 minutes

Cooking time: 6 hours

Servings: 2

Ingredients:

- ½ cup wild rice

- 1 red onion, sliced

- ½ cup brown rice

- 2 cups veggie stock

- ½ cup baby spinach

- ½ cup cherry tomatoes, halved

- 2 tablespoons pine nuts, toasted

- 1 tablespoon raisins

- 1 tablespoon chives, chopped

- 1 tablespoon dill, chopped

- ½ tablespoon olive oil

- A pinch of salt and black pepper

Directions:

1.   In your slow cooker, mix the rice with the onion, stock, and the

other ingredients, toss, put the lid on, and cook on Low for 6 hours.

2.   Divide into bowls and serve as a snack.

Nutrition:

calories 211, fat 3, carbs 3, protein 10

46. Cauliflower Spread

Preparation time: 10 minutes

Cooking time: 7 hours

Servings: 2

Ingredients:

- 1 cup cauliflower florets • 1 tablespoon mayonnaise

- ½ cup heavy cream

- 1 tablespoon lemon juice

- ½ teaspoon garlic powder

- ¼ teaspoon smoked paprika

- ¼ teaspoon mustard powder

- A pinch of salt and black pepper

Directions:

1. In your slow cooker, combine the cauliflower with the cream, mayonnaise, and the other ingredients, toss, put the lid on and cook on Low for 7 hours.

2.   Transfer to a blender, pulse well, into bowls, and serve as a

spread.

Nutrition:

47. Flavory Mushroom Dip

Preparation time: 10 minutes

Cooking time: 5 hours

Servings: 2

Ingredients:

- 4 ounces white mushrooms, chopped

- 1 eggplant, cubed

- ½ cup heavy cream

- ½ tablespoon tahini paste

- 2 garlic cloves, minced

- A pinch of salt and black pepper

- 1 tablespoon balsamic vinegar

- ½ tablespoon basil, chopped

- ½ tablespoon oregano, chopped

Directions:

1. In your slow cooker, mix the mushrooms with the eggplant, cream, and the other ingredients, toss, put the lid on and cook on High for 5 hours.

2. Divide the mushroom mix into bowls and serve as a dip.

Nutrition:

calories 189, fat 3, carbs 4, protein 3

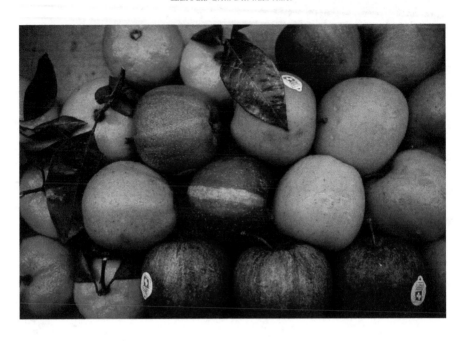

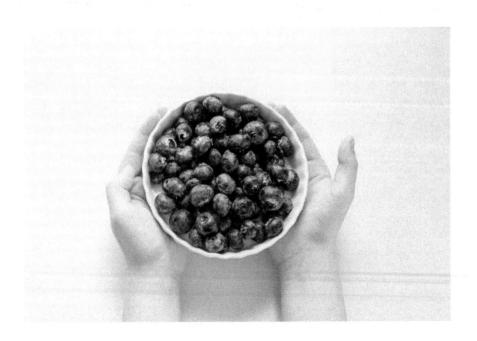

Fueling Recipes

48. Summer Bruschetta

Preparation Time: 15 minutes

Cooking Time: 3 hours

Servings: 4

Ingredients:

- Basil leaves (chopped) – 6

- Artichoke hearts (quartered) – ½ cup

- Kalamata olives (halved) – ¼ cup

- Capers – ¼ cup

- Roma tomatoes (diced) – 4

- Balsamic vinegar – 3 tablespoons

- Avocado oil – 3 tablespoons

- Onion powder – ¾ teaspoon

- Sea salt – ¾ teaspoon

- Black pepper – ½ teaspoon

- Garlic (minced) – 2 tablespoons

Directions:

1. Mix all the fixings in the slow cooker and stir mix.

2. Cook for 3 hours on high, stirring the mix after every hour.

Nutrition:

Calories: 152 Total Carbohydrate: 4 g Cholesterol: 1 mg

Total Fat: 13 g Fiber: 4 g Protein: 1 g

Sodium: 140 mg

49. Tomato Cheddar Fondue

Preparation Time: 20 minutes

Cooking Time: 30 minutes

Servings: 3-1/2 cups

Ingredients:

- 1 garlic clove, halved

- 6 medium tomatoes, seeded and diced

- 2/3 cup dry white wine

- 6 tablespoons. butter, cubed

- 1-1/2 teaspoons. dried basil

- Dash cayenne pepper

- 2 cups shredded cheddar cheese

- 1 tablespoon. all-purpose flour

- Cubed French bread and cooked shrimp

Directions:

1. Combine wine, butter, basil, cayenne and tomatoes in a large saucepan. On a medium low heat, bring mixture to a simmer, then decrease heat to low. Mix cheese with flour. Add to tomato mixture gradually while stirring after each addition until cheese is melted.

2. Pour into the fondue pot and keep warm. Enjoy with shrimp and bread cubes.

Nutrition:

Calories: 118 Total Carbohydrate: 4 g

Cholesterol: 30 mg Total Fat: 10 g

Fiber: 1 g

Protein: 4 g

50. Swiss Seafood Canapés

Preparation Time: 20 minutes

Cooking Time: 25 minutes

Servings: 4

Ingredients:

- 1 can (6 oz.) small shrimp, rinsed and drained

- 1 package (6 oz.) frozen crabmeat, thawed

- 1 cup shredded Swiss cheese

- 2 hard-boiled large eggs, chopped

- 1/4 cup finely chopped celery

- 1/4 cup mayonnaise

- 1/4 cup French salad dressing or seafood cocktail sauce

- 2 green onions, chopped

- Dash salt

- 1 loaf (16 oz.) snack rye bread

Directions:

1.   Mix the first fixings in a large bowl. Put bread on ungreased baking sheets.

2.   Broil for 1 to 2 minutes, 4 to 6-inches from the heat or until lightly browned. Flip slices over; spread 1 rounded tablespoonful of seafood mixture on each.

Nutrition:

Calories: 57   Total Carbohydrate: 5 g

Cholesterol: 22 mg   Total Fat: 3 g

Fiber: 1 g

Protein: 3 g

Conclusion

It is the last article in my series on Lean and Green Recipes. Thank you so much for sticking with me all this way, and I hope you found it helpful. I have compiled a series of useful resources at the end of this article, including some wonderful books, websites and podcasts. I can recommend readers who have more knowledge about sustainable living or cooking to interested readers. They helped me a lot over the last few years and I hope they can do the same for you too.

Lean cooking is a style of cooking that emphasizes relatively low-fat content and minimal use of oil. Lean meat, fish, vegetables and grains are cooked in the minimum amount of fat necessary to preserve them. It's not a very customizable way to cook because you can't change the fat content or oil used (you can however swap out all the lean ingredients with higher fat ones).

Green cooking is a style of cooking that emphasizes lessening the environmental impact of your meal preparation by focusing on local, seasonal produce, along with avoiding the use of processed foods or meats that have been produced overseas. As with Lean cooking, it's not very customizable since you're required to buy local and seasonal produce.

The basic idea behind Lean and Green cooking is to approach your weekly meal planning from a perspective of total calories instead of from a perspective of how many calories you are getting from fat or protein. You can use the concepts and recipes I provide to make your own lean meats and green foods, or you can improvise new things.

Because Lean and Green cooking approaches your weekly meal planning from a perspective of total calories instead of from a perspective of how many calories you are getting from fat or protein, it helps you develop a more mindful relationship with food. It's easier to overeat and to consume more calories than you need when you don't pay attention to the actual numbers of food that you're eating. Lean and Green cooking helps break this cycle and make you more aware of your relationship with food in a positive way.

It's also a very simple way to eat, once you figure out what combination of foods works best for your body. And this is where I've found the most appeal for myself personally. My body feels great when I eat a nutritious diet, but I'm also very aware of how many calories I'm eating, and simultaneously, how much fat or protein is in those calories. And if my stomach feels like it's about to boom (which it does sometimes!), I know that there's enough food in my meal that makes me satisfied and not too full.

I hope you can take some of my lessons into your own kitchen. And if you substitute a few ingredients or otherwise make adjustments to suit your tastes, feel free! After all, that's really what creating food is all about: using whatever ingredients you have for what dish you want to create. What matters is the love and care that go into it.

CPSIA information can be obtained
at www.ICGtesting.com
Printed in the USA
BVHW051102040821
613618BV00008B/91